OPENING THE DOOR

TO THE BRAIN

GRANULAR CELL NEURON MASSES

By
Hyman Olken

Olken Publications

2830 Kennedy Street, Livermore, CA 94550, U.S.A.

PREFACE

Decades ago the neurological profession started to do research of the human brain i.e., the cortex. At the outset they made a big mistake and have been doing it for decades since. The particulars of this mistake are as follows:

The human cortex is composed of two anatomical formations. One formation is composed of layers of large, pyramid cells. The other formation is composed of layers of tiny (granular) cells. The layers of granular cells are interweaved with the layers of pyramid cells.

One day in 1963 I was working on an invited paper for the Houston Neurological Symposium - a paper on the memory process in the cortex. While working on that paper I discovered this astonishing thing. In the entire neurological literature, the number of papers on the tiny granular cells were so few that you could count them on the fingers of one hand. But the papers on the large, pyramid cells could be counted by the thousands!

I realized this was a mistake and set about to correct it. This I did by writing a fundamental, basic paper on the granular cell neuron masses. This paper contained a comprehensive review of all the electronic oscillation phenomenon that occurred in the cortex. It is therefore a tremendous help in neurological research.

This paper was not presented to a neurological conference. Instead, being an electronics engineer, I presented it to an electronics engineering conference - the NAECON - National Aerospace and Electronics Engineering Conference, held in Dayton, Ohio, May 1963. They accepted the paper, it was presented at the conference, and the paper was published (that year) in the proceedings of the conference. However, neurologists do not read the technical literature of the electronics engineering profession, so that paper was, in effect, unpublished.

In 1989 I published a little book on the memory process in the human cortex and added this paper to it as an appendix. However, this resulted in very little publication in the neurological literature.

To overcome schizophrenia, epilepsy, and other ailments of the nervous system you need to understand the whole cortex, not just a half of it. To do that the neurological profession will have to become informed on the granular cell neuron formations of the cortex. This they can do by publication of my paper on the granular cell neuron masses.

To fully understand the content of this paper one must have a professional background in neurology. One must also have a Ph.D. background in electronic engineering. There are very few people with these two backgrounds. That is why it has been extremely difficult to get this paper published. So I have decided to publish it in the focus of this little book.

In short, to overcome schizophrenia and epilepsy, one has to understand the whole cortex, not just one half of it. And this can be managed by making my paper on the granular cell neurons an integral part of the neurological literature.

GRANULAR CELL NEURON MASSES

CONTENTS

INTRODUCTION

The coherent action of large masses of neurons as a single, powerful electrical unit has been known for a long time. This phenomenon occurs in all parts of the nervous system -- in the spinal chord, in the subcortical centers, and in the brain -- and it is manifested in several different forms: as a steady, normal activity of the brain, called "brain waves"; as a response to electrical or sensory stimulation, in an effect similar to the "ringing" of an electrical circuit, called "evoked potentials"; and, under pathological conditions, as a tidal wave of electrical activity which engulfs most or the whole of the nervous system, and is known as "epileptic fits".

Neurophysiologists have found many remarkable correlations between these forms of coherent neuron mass action and human intellectual activity. For example, the different types of brain waves (alpha, beta, delta and theta) correlate closely with different stages of mental development and activity (ref. 1). However, our understanding of these correlations, and hence our insight into how the brain works as a thinking mechanism, has so far been limited because the prevailing theories of coherent neuron mass action do not provide an adequate physical explanation of the phenomenon. An attempt is therefore made in this paper to develop a more comprehensive physical explanation. This has been done by utilizing a long-known principle of electronic engineering and combining it with new knowledge gained from recent advances in the field or neurophysiology.

The coherent electrical activity of large neuron populations takes place predominantly in the cortex, so this paper will be confined to the consideration of this phenomenon as it occurs in the cortex only. To treat it for the other nervous system areas where it also occurs -- in the subcortical centers and spinal chord -- would make this presentation too lengthy and complex.

ANATOMICAL BACKGROUND

To gain an insight into the physical mechanism of coherent electrical activity of neuron masses one must keep in mind a few of the salient facts of neuroanatomy.

The human nervous system is made up of two principal types of components. One is a nerve cell with a long extension, called the axon, which transmits an electrical impulse over a considerable distance through this axon. They are the type shown at the left of figure 73 in Lorente' de No's classic chapter on the cerebral cortex in reference 2. The other major component are the tiny cells called granular or stellate cells, in which the axon branches all lie close to the cell body and fall within the field of the receiving end of the nerve cell, called the dendrite tree. These are indicated on the right of the same figure in reference 2.

The most significant feature of the nervous system anatomy, as far as coherent neuron mass action is concerned, is that the long-axon or transmission nerve cells do not transmit directly to one another, but always go through intervening large masses of these granular cells. Thus the central part of the spinal chord comprises one huge mass of these granular cells over its entire length (fig. 5, ref. 3, and fig. 2, ref. 30) and the peripheral nerves which come into or go out of the chord to all parts of the body all connect to each other through this huge granular cell mass, as is also shown in figure 24 of reference 4. In the brain, the incoming and outgoing transmission nerves connect to each other through similar large granular cell masses formed in horizontal layers in the cortex, as shown in figures 69 and 70, also in Lorente' de No's chapter (ref. 2). In the subcortical centers, located between the brain and spinal chord, the transmission neurons likewise connect through large granular cell masses that occur in huge clumps called nuclei, as shown in figure 5A of reference 5.

The characteristics and functions of the long, transmission type nerve cells have been pretty well explored and are quite well understood, especially since the development of microelectrodes that penetrate directly into the cell (fig. 2, ref. 6).

It is now widely realized that the long-axon neurons constitute three basic functional types: 1) transducers, called sensory neurons, which convert a sensation (pressure, temperature, etc.) into a train of electrical pulses; 2) relay neurons, which transmit these pulses from one point to another; and 3) effectors, which convert the electrical pulse into a muscle movement or a gland secretion. These are shown in figure 1 of reference 7. The short-axon neurons have not been so intensively studied and their characteristics are less well understood.

Another highly significant anatomical feature is the very peculiar anatomical formation of the cortex. It is made up of massive horizontal layers of granular cells, called also stellate cells, sandwiched in between layers of large pyramid cells (fig. 2, Plate XI, ref 8 and plate 8, p. 30, ref. 10). The stellate cells have axons and dendrites coming out in all directions from the cell body, and these branch in all directions, in the area very close to the cell body, as seen in figure 73, reference 2 and in plate 5, reference 10. The pyramid cells also have a unique but different shape. The cell body is distinctly triangular or pyramidal in shape. One massive dendrite stem projects upward from the apex of the pyramid, hence is called the apical dendrite tree. Two extensive dendrite arborizations also extend out horizontally from each of the two angles at the base of the pyramidal body, hence are called basilar dendrites. This unique configuration (fig. 3, ref. 9 and fig. 4, ref. 30), is remarkably consistent throughout a wide variety of these pyramid cells that occur in the cortical layers.

Usually a single axon extends out from the base of the pyramidal cell body and reaches down vertically, with horizontal branches extending outward along its length. In a considerable proportion of pyramid cells the horizontal branches curve back upwards. These are called recurrent axon branches (fig. 3, ref. 10). The pyramidal axon branches and the basilar dendrite trees form feltworks of fibers (called "plexuses") which are interlaced through the different cell layers (fig. 75, ref. 1, and fig. 210, ref. 3).

The extensive neuron connections to the cortex enter the inner surface of the cortex as a forest of heavy fibers which extend radially, and through the cell and plexus layers, toward the outer surface of the cortex (plate 2, ref. 12). Another important point is that all axons, both those coming into and out of the cortex, normally have thick myelin sheaths or coverings which increase the speed of electrical impulse transmission along the axon, but inside the cortex they have no such sheaths. Thus cortical neurons have the dendrites and axons in close contact with one another. Finally, this complex formation of cells and fibers is suspended in a mass of glia cells (plate 7, ref. 13), which act as a supporting medium for the architectural arrangement and act as metabolic links connecting the intensely active neurons with their source of nourishment, the interlaced network of capillary blood vessels. A rough idea of the whole physical conglomeration is provided by plate 6 of ref. 14.

One other anatomical feature to be kept in mind is that the formation of cells into layers, and the interlacing of the cell layers with dendrite and axon plexuses, is consistent throughout the cortex, but the thicknesses of the layers and their grouping in a particular area vary considerably in different cortical regions. Generally, as seen in figure 1 in the sensory (audio and visual) input areas the layers are distinct and the granular and pyramid layers alternate; in the motor region, which controls the skeletal musculature, there is a heavy concentration of large pyramid cells, heavily interspersed with granular cells; and in the frontal regions, believed to control higher mental capabilities, the granular cells concentration is predominant and is interspersed with pyramid cells.

PREVAILING THEORIES

The theories of the coherent electrical behavior presently widely held are mainly variations of two classical concepts which rest on divergent interpretations of the role of this peculiar anatomical structure of the cortex. One is the "reverberating chain" concept propounded by Lorente' de No and based on his classic anatomical studies of the cortex (ref. 2). This theory holds that the neuron masses, such as the regions of the cortex, are made up of small local neuron clusters in which a few long-axon neurons are connected, by interspersed short-axon neurons, to form closed loops or chains. A stimulus input to one link in the chain is transmitted around the chain, then continues to circulate or reverberate around the closed loop. This is illustrated in figure 74 of his classic chapter on the cerebral cortex (ref. 2).

The other concept is that of "random networks" which is championed by Sholl (ref. 15) and W. Gray Walter (ref. 1) and is based on the work of leading experimenters such as Adrian (ref. 16), Bishop (ref. 17), and Bremer (ref. 18). This theory holds that in the large neuron masses each neuron forms random connections with a great many others, hence stimulation is transferred between one large group of neurons and another by connections formed between them, at the moment, on a probableistic or statistical basis. As so emphatically stated by Sholl (ref. 15), "Histological studies show that no theory, mathematical or other, relying on specific circuits can be maintained. The alternative approach must depend on statistical considerations in which the connections of individual neurons are of less concern and the connectivity of the neuronal aggregate is studied".

THE MULTIVIBRATOR CONCEPT

The electronic engineering principle that helps explain the neuron mass action in these cortical formations is that of the multivibrator circuit. This is commonly considered as a relaxation oscillator only, but the circuit concept is much broader than that. Basically the multivibrator comprises two stages of resistance-coupled amplified with appropriate feed back from one stage to the other (fig. 18-9, ref. 19). Therefore, if the circuit parameters are right and there is little feed back, this 2-stage unit operates as an amplifier and transfers or relays an input signal, but in magnified form (fig. 3-1a, ref. 20). But if the circuit parameters and feed back are changed it can function as a relaxation type self-oscillator (fig. 18-10, ref. 21). Still other combinations of circuit parameters in each resistance amplifier stage, and another value of feed back between them will make this 2-stage unit a "synchronous" or "lock-in" oscillator which will oscillate at the frequency of an input driving pulse (fig. 18-15, ref. 22). Finally, still further change in circuit parameters within each amplifier stage and still another value of feed back will make the 2-stage combination operate as the familiar flip-flop, in which the output voltage swings back and forth from one polarity to another (figs. 8.1 and 8.2, ref. 23).

The important point here is that we have an electrical unit which will shift from one to another of four distinctly different modes of operation (amplification, self-oscillation, lock-in oscillation, and flip-flop) without change from one type of circuit to another -- merely by changes of internal parameters of the same basic circuit.

This helps us to understand the physical mechanism of coherent electrical activity in neuron masses in this way. One ordinarily thinks of coherence neuron masses only as oscillators which generate those periodic electrical oscillations known as brain waves. But if we study these spontaneous regional electrical activities more closely, we find that this self-oscillation is only part of a much broader picture of electrical activity in cortical regional cell masses. For, in addition to self-oscillation, localized groups of cortical cells can also function as lock-in oscillators. That is, the regional cell mass will oscillate at the frequency of a received (driving) input (ref. 24). Furthermore, a regional cell mass may operate as a flip-flop. That is, an incoming pulse can shift the mass from one state of dc polarization to the opposite and back again (ref. 25). Finally, local cell aggregates in the cortex will act as a relay or amplifier. That is, the incoming pulse is passed on to other parts of the cortex, but with considerable increase in intensity; in other works, with amplification (ref. 26).

Just as in the case of self-oscillation, the same things may occur in these other modes of cell-mass operation. That is, when functioning as an amplifier, flip-flop, or lock-in oscillator, the regional aggregate of cells can also expand or contract, or spread from one area of the cortex to another (ref. 7).

Another major and important part of this picture is that the expansion or contraction of a local aggregate will be largely influenced by changes in metabolic conditions in that region (ref. 28). Also, metabolic changes may cause a regional cell aggregate to shift from one of these modes of operation to another -- say from flip-flop to lock-in oscillation, or any other shift from one mode to another (ref. 29).

In short, the electrical units formed by coherent neuron masses can operate in any one of the four modes of multivibrator operation (amplification, self-oscillation, lock-in oscillation and flip-flop), and can shift from one of these modes to another <u>without changes in neuron circuits</u> merely by changes of metabolic conditions, which in effect determine the internal circuit parameters of the multivibrator unit. Some changes of circuitry within the coherent neuron mass do take place, by increased length and heavier branching of neurons as they grow (fig. 4, ref. 30), but this is a long term affair.

Hence, the basic mechanism underlying coherence neuron mass action must be that of two electrical energy transfer units coupled together with suitable feed back between them, like the two amplifier stages of the multivibrator. Such a mechanism has been discovered recently by Dr. Holgar Hyden in the interaction between the cortical pyramid cells and the glia cells which surround them

THE NEURON-GLIA TISSUE MULTIVIBRATOR

Dr. Hyden's thesis has been that the nerve cells in the cortex are all embedded in large numbers of glia cells. Hence these glia cells must play an important part in the operation of the neuron masses of the cortex, among which the glia cells are so heavily interspersed. A picture of this glia-neuron formation is given in his figure 2 in reference 31.

After many years of brilliant investigation which involved the development of electronic experimental equipment that permits precise, rapid, chemical analysis of nerve cells and their adjoining glia cells, Dr. Hyden came to this conclusion (ref. 31): "The experimental evidence indicates a very close relationship between the neuron and its glia, the latter apparently constituting an effective feed back mechanism coordinating the electrical and biochemical processes in the neuron".

(Incidentally, there is a very clear and comprehensive summary of all of Dr. Hyden's work in the recent article by him in the British magazine Endeavour for October 1962. This article summarizes his development of electronic devices and lab techniques for these micro-analyses, as well as his discoveries and conclusions about the chemical interactions between nerve cells and their related glia.)

Specifically, it appears from Dr. Hyden's work that the cortical pyramid nerve cells and its adjoining glia form a 2-stage energy transfer unit, with appropriate feed back between the two stages, like the 2-stage amplifier combination in the multivibrator. Obviously, then, if metabolic conditions should change for the pyramidal neuron and its related glia, say by increase or decrease of blood supply to the local cortical region, this would be equivalent to changing the circuit parameters of the two amplifier stages of the multivibrator circuit or the degree of feed back between them. We should therefore expect metabolic changes to cause shifts of cortical neuron-glia masses from one to another of their modes of electrical operation (amplification, flip-flop, self-oscillation, lock-in oscillation).

We can therefore picture the pyramid cells of the cortex, with their surrounding glia cells, as forming a massive tissue which will operate as a powerful electrical unit in one of the four modes of multivibrator operation, depending on the metabolic conditions present. Such an electrical unit -- on the basis of its anatomical features -- could well be continuously active, particularly in the self-oscillation mode; and would probably be highly stable, because of the constancy of the metabolic conditions in the cortex; hence it would account for the alpha waves in the cortex which are (in most people) constantly present, have remarkable frequency stability (ref. 32), and are of such powerful amplitude that they show up, through the skull, as measurable brain waves over the scalp (ref. 1).

Should this pyramidal neuron-glia tissue, acting as a multivibrator, be the factor which provides the basic driving force in the coherent electrical activity of cortical neuron aggregates, as just hypothesized, then the massive stimulation inputs from the different sense organs would constitute an electrical activity overlayed on top of it. This would account readily for the "blocking" of the alpha brain waves which take place in many people when their eyes are opened and a number of other correlations, already found, between the brain waves and learning, conditioning, and other mental activities (ref. 33).

THE GRANULAR CELL TISSUE

Although the pyramid cells and their adjoining glia form the principal tissue in the cortex, the granular cell mass also comprises an important anatomical formation (fig. 1, ref. 39). These cells, on the basis of their physical features alone, will have these electrical characteristics:

a) Self excitation. Since the dendrite tree and axon arborization are both extensive and distributed near each other, close to the cell body, there will be heavy feed back between the input and output ends of each cell. This will give each cell a strong tendency to act as a self-excited, single stage multivibrator (ref. 1).

b) Similar Characteristics. The granular cells correspond closely in size and configuration, so will tend to have similar electrical behavior characteristics. They will therefore be responsive in large numbers, or "resonant", to a narrow range of input stimulus frequencies.

c) Close Coupling. Being close to one another and with the axons and dendrite fibers of one cell heavily interlocked with those of another, the granular cells will act as very closely coupled electrical units. Hence they will tend to act in the old familiar electrical phenomenon best known by its German name of "Ziehen", in which closely coupled oscillators of nearly the same resonant frequency "pull" each other into a common mode of oscillation.

We can therefore expect the granular cell tissue to:

1) Act as a powerful relaxation oscillator, due to the heavy feed back between each cell's axon and dendrite trees.

2) Be sharply resonant to a narrow range of input stimulus frequencies, due to the cells' very similar electrical characteristics.

3) Take some time for oscillation of the entire mass to build up, due to the time required for the individual cells to lock into step with one another by the "Ziehen" effect. Also, for this reason, the build-up would be confined to a local area, where the granular cells are heavily concentrated.

In a remarkable informative recent paper, W. Gray Walter points out how, with micro-probes placed within the cortex, just such coherent mass characteristics have been observed. These are shown in figures 7-3 (powerful osc.), 7-1 (resonance), and 7-2 (duration of build-up), respectively, of reference 34.

One can therefore picture the coherent neuron aggregate activity of the cortex as the resultant of two separate coherent mass activities interacting with one another. One is the coherent activity of the neuron-glia tissue multivibrator, which produces a powerful, continuous, electrical activity that underlies brain waves; another is the coherent activity of the granular cell mass, which builds up to a powerful oscillatory unit if stimulated for a long enough time, by input stimuli of a narrow frequency band, and which is confined spatially to where the granular cells are concentrated.

INTERACTIONS BETWEEN TISSUES

Ordinarily we would expect these two tissues to interact in a manner depending on the sensory input stimulation and the prevailing metabolic conditions. Walter has shown that this is the case, the over-all effect being a series of characteristic waves in the visual cortex in an effect similar to the "ringing" of an electrical circuit and is known as "after effect" (fig. 7-7, ref. 34). However, under pathological conditions, such as epilepsy, the driving by the glia-neuron tissue becomes so powerful that the granular cell mass of a very large brain area becomes thrown into oscillation. Recordings from inside the brain for this condition show that it starts out with the wave form characteristic of alpha waves (fig. 8A, ref. 35), but soon builds up into a very powerful, smooth saw tooth wave "envelope" that is to be expected from a a huge mass of small oscillators locked in step with one another (fig. 8B, 8C, ref. 35). In other words, in this case the driving granular cell mass is set into such powerful oscillation by the neuron-glia tissue "driver" that the driver becomes locked into step with natural oscillation pattern of the driven unit. This continues until metabolic exhaustion of the tissues stops the powerful oscillations and the whole system reverts to the initial wave form of the neuron-glia tissue's normal activity (fig. 8D, ref. 35).

Considering the lower intensity level of interacting activity between the neuron-glia and the granular cells tissues, it is reasonable to venture a guess that, during response to a normal sensory input, an elementary unit of the neuron-glia tissue may become "occluded" with a cluster of surrounding granular cells to form a sharply tuned memory recording element or "memory trace" which is particularly responsive to, and hence can be easily re-excited or recalled, when a later stimulus of the same frequency arrives. This would account for the "distributed" formation of memory traces or memory storage that is known to occur, particularly from the work of Lashley (ref. 36).

The neuron-glia and granular cell tissues are the major ones in the cortex, but a variety of other types exist. Sholl has shown that the pyramid and granular (stellate) cells in the cortex are of seven principal types which differ mainly in the direction and extent of their axon and dendrite arborizations (fig 3, ref. 37). He shows how the relative concentrations of the different types can be determined in a particular region (fig. 4, ref. 38). From this diagram it is seen that the type of cell more heavily concentrated in a particular area forms a particular tissue. Lorente' de No's classic chapter (ref. 2) shows the different types of tissues and the available interconnections between them. One can therefore form a table of the tissues present in the cortex, defining for each tissue: a) the predominant cell types composing it; and b) its tie-in to other cortical cell masses (layers), hence its tissue-interconnecting function. For example, in the visual cortex, there is a layer of smaller pyramid cells above the granular cell layer, which pyramids send dendrite trees to interconnect mainly with one another and with granular cell layer below. One would therefore expect the small pyramid layer to be driven by the granular cell layer. Also, these small pyramids send axons predominantly to the inner (large) pyramid layers of the cortex. Hence this small pyramid tissue would interact with, and thus tie together, the granular cell layer with the lower pyramid layers of the cortex.

W. G. Walter, in the above mentioned article (ref. 34) has mentioned the possibility that the coherent action of neuron masses in a particular cortical locality may act as a "gating" mechanism which controls the transference of neuronal activity to other cortical regions, and this "gating" function may be the means for organizing the pattern of activity that goes on in different cortical areas during a particular mental or intelligence function (ref. 24). I would therefore venture the guess that it is the interaction between these different tissues which determines this gating action, and thereby sets the pattern of activity in different cortical areas that underlies a particular mental function.

SUMMARY

To summarize, we can conceive of the cortex as made up of different tissues, each tissue made up of predominantly one type of nerve cell. Each tissue can act as a multivibrator unit, and can shift from one of the four modes of multivibrator operation to another depending on internal metabolic conditions. The four modes are: self-oscillation, lock-in or synchronous oscillator operation, flip-flop operation and relay or amplification operation. Response of a tissue to sensory inputs is overlaid on top of these four basic states of activity. Interaction between tissues may serve as a "gating" function which permits transfer of neuronal activity from one cortical region to another. This "gating" function is very likely the mechanism which patterns the particular organizations of activity in different cortical regions that underlies particular human mental functions.

ILLUSTRATIONS

Fig. 1 Different anatomical formations in different regions of the cortex. (A) prefrontal cortex; (B) motor cortex; (C) sensory (visual) cortex. (Adopted from A. W. Campbell, "Histological Studies on the Localization of Cerebral Function", 1905. Courtesy Cambridge Univ. Press.)

REFERENCES

Ref. 1 W. Grey Walter, "Intrinsic Rhythms of the Brain", Handbook of Physiology, Section I, Neurophysiology, Vol I, American Physiology Society, Washington, D.C.; 1959; pp. 279-298.

Ref. 2 R. Lorente′ de No, "Cerebral Cortex: Architecture, Intercortical Connections, Motor Projections", in J. F. Fulton, Physiology of the Nervous System, 3d ed., Ch. XV, pp. 288-330, Oxford, N.Y.: 1949.

Ref. 3 O. Larson, "Textbook of Neuroanatomy and the Sense Organs", D. Appleton - Century Co., N.Y., 1939; fig. 57, p. 68.

Ref. 4 Hyman S. Rubinstein, "The Study of the Brain", Grune & Stratton, N.Y., 1953; fig. 24, p. 69.

Ref. 5 C. A. Terzuolo and W. R. Adey, "Sensorimotor Cortical Activities", Ch. XXXIII, pp. 797-835, Handbook of Physiology, Vol. II (ref. 1) 1960; fig. 5A, p. 819.

Ref. 6 Wilfrid Roll, "Electrophysiology of a Dendritic Neuron Model", in Biophysical Journal, Vol. 2, No. 2, pt. 2, March 1962, pp. 145-167; fig. 2, p. 147.

Ref. 7 David Bodian, "The Generalized Vertebrate Neuron", Science, Vol. 137, pp. 323-326, Aug. 3, 1962; fig. 1, p. 325.

Ref. 8 A. W. Campbell, "Histological Studies on the Localization of Cerebral Function", Cambridge Univ. Press, 1905; plate XI, fig. 2.

Ref. 9 R. Cooper, "Brain Mechanisms: Natural and Artificial", Research (London), Aug. 1961, pp. 329-336; fig. 3, p 331.

Ref. 10 D. A. Sholl, "Organization of the Cerebral Cortex", John Wiley, N.y., 1956; fig. 3, p. 45.

Ref. 11 R. Lorente' de No; (ref. 2); fig. 75, p. 310.

Ref. 12 D. A. Sholl (ref. 10), plate 2, p. 4.

Ref. 13 D. A. Sholl (ref. 10), plate 7, p. 17.

Ref. 14 D. A. Sholl (ref. 10), plate 6, p. 15.

Ref. 15 D. A. Sholl (ref. 10), p. 102.

Ref. 16 E. D. Adrian, "The Physical Background of Perception", Claredon Press, Oxford, 1947.

Ref. 17 G. H. Bishop, and M. H. Clare, Journal of Neurophysiology, vol 15, p. 201, 1952.

Ref. 18 F. Bremer, "Considerations Sur L'origine Et La Nature Des "Ondes" Cerebrales, Encephalography and Clinical Neurophysiology, Vol. I, p. 177-193, 1949.

Ref. 19 F. E. Terman, "Electronic and Radio Engineering", pp. 625-634; 4th ed., 1955, McGraw-Hill, N.Y.; fig. 18-9, p. 626.

Ref. 20 Electronic Designers' Handbook, R. W. Landee, D. C. Davis and A. P. Albrecht, editors, McGraw-Hill, N.Y., 1957, fig. 3-1a, p. 3-3.

Ref. 21 F. E. Terman, (ref. 19), fig. 18-10, p. 626.

Ref. 22 F. E. Terman (ref. 19), fig. 18-15, p. 631.

Ref. 23 Electronic Designers' Handbook (ref. 20), fig. 8.1, p. 8-2 and 8.2, p. 8-3.

Ref. 24 R. Cooper and A. C. Mundy Castle, "Spatial and Temporal Characteristics of the Alpha Rhythm: A Toposcopic Analysis", Electro-encephalography and Clinical Neurophysiology, vol. 12, pp. 153-165, 1960; p. 162.

Ref. 25 B. D. Burns, "Some Properties of Isolated Cerebral Cortex in the Unanesthetized Cat." Journal of Physiology, vol. 112, p. 156-175, 1951.

Ref. 26 W. Gray Walter (ref. 32), p. 243.

Ref. 27 R. Cooper and A. C. Mundy-Castle (ref. 24), p. 161.

Ref. 28 W. Grey Walter (ref. 32), p. 249.

Ref. 29 W. Grey Walter (ref. 32), p. 255.

Ref. 30 S. A. Sarkisov, "The Functional Interpretation of Certain Morphological Structures of Cortex of the Brain in the Evolutionary Aspect". pp. 81-87, in Structure and Function of the Cerebral Cortex, ed. by D. B. Tower; Proceedings of the Amsterdam Internat. Meeting on Neurophysiol; 1959; D. Van Norstrand, N.Y., 1961.

Ref. 31 Holgar Hyden, "The Neuron and Its Glia -- A Biochemical and Functional Unit", Endeavour (London), vol. XXI, No. 83-84, Oct. 1962, p. 144-155; fig. 2, p. 147.

Ref. 32 W. Grey Walter, "Oscillatory Activity in the Nervous System", ch. 7, pp. 222-257, in Neural Physiopathology, R. C. Grenell, ed., Harper & Row, N.Y., 1962; p. 246.

Ref. 33 R. Galambos and C. T. Morgan, "The Neural Basis of Learning", ch. LXI, pp. 1471-1499, Vol. III, Handbook of Physiology (ref. 1).

Ref. 34 W. Grey Walter (ref. 32), figures 7-1, p. 299; 7-2, p. 230; 7-3, p. 232; 7-7, p. 242.

Ref. 35 A. A. Ward, Jr., "Epilepsy", pp. 137-186 in International Review of Neurobiology, vol. 3, C. C.

Pfeiffer & J. R. Smythies, editors, Academic Press, N.Y., 1961; figs. 8A, p. 170, 8B, p. 171, 8C, p. 172.

Ref. 36 K. S. Lashley, "In Search of the Engram", in Physiological Mechanisms of Animal Behavior, Symposium of Society for Experimental Biology, Vol. IV, pp. 454-482, Academic Press, N.Y., 1950.

Ref. 37 D. A. Sholl (ref. 10), fig. 3, p. 45.

Ref. 38 D. A. Sholl (ref. 10), fig. 4, p. 49.

Ref. 39 N. L. Mitra, "Quantitative Analysis of Cell Types in Mammalian Neo Cortex", Journal of Anatomy (London), vol. 89, pp. 467-483, Jan-Oct. 1955; fig. 1, p. 472.

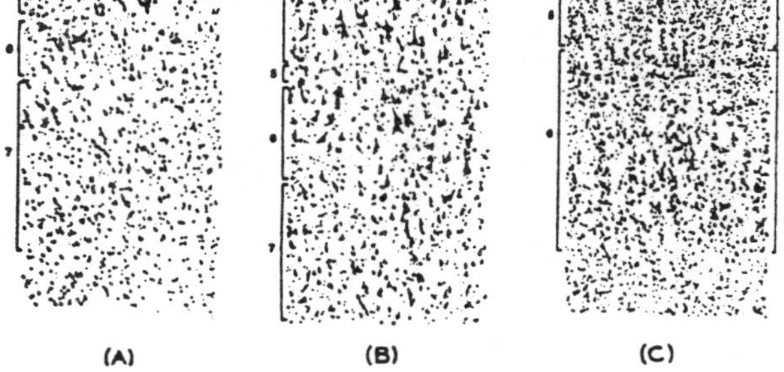

FIGURE 1

For a good discussion of the action of the nerve cells as electrical oscillators, in all parts of the brain, see the article by R. R. Linas, The Intrinsic Electro-Physiological Properties of Mamalian Neurons: Insights into Central Nervous System Function. SCIENCE, vol. 242, 23 Dec. 1988, pp. 1654-1664.